You Too Can Be A Survivor!

Mrs. Phyllis Alexander

To order additional copies of this book, contact:
Xlibris Corporation
1-888-795-4274
www.Xlibris.com
Orders@Xlibris.com
69300

YOU TOO CAN BE A SURVIVOR!!!!!!

Dedications

This book is dedicated to my wonderful husband, Dwight Alexander, for he is the person that suggested that I tell my story. I kept telling him that I wanted to do something that would help women and men, yes men do get Breast Cancer I thought, if I could help save just one life, then my life on earth would be more meaningful. I would also like to dedicate this book to all my family and friends that died from cancer This also goes out to those who succumb to Breast Cancer, across the world.

A SPECIAL DEDICATICATION TO MY AUNT LOUISE:

Louise Watson: A special thanks to my dear aunt that prayed with me through my battle and also supported me. She herself is now battling cancer, and my prayers go out to her. She gives so much of herself and wants nothing in return. God Bless You Wesse!

ACKNOWLEDGMENTS

First, to my Lord and Savior without whom, none of this would have been possible. For he gave me the courage and inspiration to write this book and to make all women aware of early detection, but especially African-American women whose incidence of death from breast cancer is higher than that of other women. Therefore, since I am a breast cancer survivor, I would like to spread the word, and encourage other patients to fight and become survivors too. Please don't linger, do your self-examinations and get those mammograms.

DWIGHT ALEXANDER: I love you before the diagnosis, and I truly love you now, for God sent me an angel to see me through.

WILLIAM AND MARY JACKSON: To my parents whose love and support kept me going. You are the best, I often told you I couldn't have asked for better parents, I will love you always.

CAROL BERRY: My oldest sister who was the first person I called, she calmed me down and had the faith that I would make it. When I was a teenager I was glad to have her to talk to and I still am today. Thanks sis.

SHARON MOORE: My sister, who went with me to my radiation consultation so that I could start my treatment, she also bought me hats to make me feel better when my hair started coming out. Thanks for being there.

CATHY TODD: My youngest sister, who also went with me to my consultation, she also brought me hats and little things that made me feel a lot better about myself. THANKS CATHY.

WILLIAM JACKSON JR.: My brother, who kept me laughing, so that I could get through those really rough times. He teased me constantly and I knew he was also covering his own pain, as he watched me go through mine. Brother I know you would do anything for me, and I will always be there for you. I Love You.

ELAINE BAIN: To my best friend and Roadie, you were always there for me and I will never forget you. She came almost every day to see how I was doing and if she could do anything for me. She herself had been through chemotheraphy and would suggest things that she did for her nausea. She even cut my hair down so that it would be less dramatic when it all started coming out. She shared with me later, years later that as she was cutting my hair the tears were rolling down her face and so that I would not see her crying she went into my kitchen to get herself together. She felt so bad that her best friend was now going through exactly the same pain of fighting a deadly disease. What a friend I have I hope everyone going through this has a friend like my Elaine. Love You.

CLAUDELL ALEXANDER: My brother-in-law, who also gave me support and would call me all the time to see how I was doing. When I told him I was writing a book he gave the utmost support. Telling me, "I know you can do it." He also sent me his sons's typewriter until I brought my own. He even threw in a tape recorder. Thanks Beaver.

DR. ANNIE WANG: Pediatric doctor at the clinic I worked at before I took sick, 3001 Walnut.

In march of 1995, when I returned to work after all my treatments were done, it was Dr. Wang that suggested they give me a welcome back, birthday party combined. I had written a letter to the staff thanking them for their cards and most of all their prayers. As it was being read the entire lunch room was choked up with tears, me included, I stated in the letter how I felt about GOD allowing me to return to work and to friends that I had missed greatly. When it was finished being read, she came up to me and asked me if I had ever thought about writing. I told her that I loved to write and always did, and she replied that I should seriously think about writing something because I write so very well. Thanks for the encouragement.

TO MY COWORKERS AT THE CLINIC: I wish to extend my sincere thanks to all of my true friends you know who you are, for standing behind me through all my trials and tribulations and especially my most recent respiratory problems. I enjoyed working with all the friends that supported me when I was down. You will be sincerely missed.

DEBORAH VEASLEY; The Manager at the clinic when I was going through my bout. She always teased me about writing notes to her, it was because I arrived at work at 6:30 am and I usually remained in my office until lunchtime, at which time she could be anywhere in the clinic. We hardly ever crossed paths unless she needed something from my department. See Deb, my writing notes paid off.

DR. PATRICIA FORD: JUST THANKS. she is my Oncologist and a very very good one at that.

STAFF AT GRADUATE'S HEMOTOLOGY-ONCO-LOGY; Thanks for all your support.

DR. WILLIAM KATRINS: my Podiatrist, my Friend. I want to express my sincere gratitude for always listening to me, even when you were dealing with your loss. This proves that love comes in all colors, and ours just happen to be vanilla and chocolate. Thanks

DR. M. CALEB: Thanks for believing me when others thought I was crazy. You are an extremely gifted doctor and your patients are very lucky to have such a good

ALLERGIST/ASTHMA doctor to take care of them. Thanks for finding one of the causes for my breathing problems and suggesting I get out of medical records and for treating me with compassion.

ACKNOWLEDGEMENTS

REVEREND AND MRS. HURST
MARIE AND HENRY COLEMAN
VIOLA BINGHAM
MARY JAMES
TIJUANA HURST
RONALD JAMES
ELAINE JENKINS
RACHAEL JENKINS
ANITA JUSTIS
PAULA JOHNSON
LISA JOHNSON
CRAIG AND DIMPLES DUREN
ROBERT DUREN (GATOR)
DENNIS AND CHARLENE DUREN
TRACY ESTES
TRACY RAY
JAMES AND EVON SUTTON
JUDY MCKEATHAN
JOANNE JOHNSON
MARVA HORTON (THANKS FOR THE ANGELS)
CAROL WEST
CHARLOTTE ELLIS (THANKS FOR THE ANGELS AND THE BREAST CANCER PIN)

DR. HELENE CASSELLI (MY PCP AND MY FRIEND)
NANCY HERBST (THANKS FOR YOUR HELP,
DURING THAT SEVERE ASTHMA ATTACK)
HENRY COLEMAN JR. (CALLED OFTEN)
DR. GARY (PEDS DIRECTOR I WORKED FOR)
DANIELLE JACKSON (CAME AND CALLED
  ALWAYS)
STAFF AT DR. MONTIERO'S OFFICE (THANKS)
CAROL BLUE (GOOD FRIEND)
LEON GLOVER (GOOD FRIEND)

Note To My Readers

Dear readers, I would like to share with you what I shared with my mom shortly after being diagnosed with breast cancer. I am a catholic woman, who went to twelve years of catholic school graduating from St. Maria Goretti High School in Philadelphia. So I'm pretty well informed about religion. As a young person I drifted away from church, saying to my mom that I'm old enough to make my own choices. I attended only at Christmas Eve and maybe Easter, many of you can identify with that. Monday through Friday I worked at my job, but the weekends belonged to me. I figured I was single at the time so what did I have to stay home for This continued up until I met my husband. All I really wanted was to be in a caring and loving relationship. I come from a big family and never wanted to be alone. My cousin and I drifted in and out of relationships looking for love and commitment, which I believe we finally found. Praise the Lord.

To this day I really believe that God said "HOLD IT PHYLLIS, you have to give me RECOGNITION". When I was first diagnosed, I cried out, "WHY ME, what have I done so bad? I'm a good person, I help people, I give to the homeless, sponsor a child from Africa and her village, and have been doing so for many years, trying to give back.' God I am too young to die, I've just met the man that I've been praying for, and now I die, why, why, why? But now that God has healed me both Physically and Spiritually I now see HIS purpose. I was made to open my eyes, really open my eyes to see God Loves me, and was saving my soul as well as my life. This was the beginning of my trial and tribulations and I knew that he would guide me through.

How many of you can say that the LORD actually touched your life and gave you such a profound sense of being born again. I now attend church on a regular basis and look forward to praising the LORD. My brother will say, there goes Rev. Ike, he teases me when I start to talk about what the LORD has done for me, because before this renewal, to him I was his party sister and it must seem strange to hear me talk about the LORD.

I also shared with my mother what I believed my purpose in life was, because prior to my diagnosis I really didn't know why I was here. I come from a large family of women, who are very fertile and didn't understand why God hadn't blessed me with children also. I often would say to my mom, I wonder why? She replied, "Phyllis honestly mommy doesn't know, but I believe God will let you know someday. You were right mom, He did.

The Holidays were very tough for me, I would watch all my sisters rushing around getting ready for Santa Clause, and there I sat with my dad and mom trying to pretend that I was also happy, and that I was glad it was Christmas. But deep down inside I hated to see it come for again I would not have any children to prepare for My mother recently told me she felt guilty, being my mom, that is was something she had done, I said, oh no mom, it had nothing to do with you or I, it was the Lord's will. She went on to say that she and my sisters knew why, after a certain time on Christmas day I would have to leave. It was just to hard to see all the kids with their gifts and their parents so proud. At home I used to cry out, 'Lord, if you didn't want me to have children, then why am I here? I thought that part of being a woman was bearing children, and for years I didn't want to go out with my sister's on Mother's Day, because people would say, "Phyllis your not a mother what are you celebrating? These were some of the things I had to deal with spiritually, before I could be at peace with myself.

Now I know what my purpose is for being on this earth, it is to help other Breast Cancer patients, to also believe they too can make it. I'm also trying to get with another breast cancer survivor who also started a program called WOMAN of FAITH and HOPE, which is a self help group for women with breast cancer to Enlighten, Empower and Encourage. This program is religiously oriented and believing in religion and having hope, got me through this difficult time.

TRIALS AND TRIBULATION

THE FOLLOWING IS MY STORY:

My life was as normal as any other single woman, working and coming home to an empty house, grabbing a sandwich, watching a little television and then going to bed to get ready for the next work day. I was tired of this routine so I continued to pray and ask the LORD to please send someone loving and kind into my life. The men that I had met prior to this were unreal, they were selfish and insensitive. So in April of 1993 my best friend and Roadie, Elaine, who I believe was also single at the time, were walking past my aunt and uncle's block. As we approached the step there sat along with them the man I would later marry. He asked my aunt to introduce me to him, which she did. He said to her, "where have you been keeping this fine thing" and he went on to ask for my phone number, but we were in a hurry, I told my aunt to give it to him, and the very next day he called me and the rest as they say is history.

Within months we were living together, not proud of that, but I didn't want him to get away. I had never met such a caring and helpful human being, my immediate family will attest to that. I knew that GOD had truly answered my prayers. My luck was changing, I was happy for the first time in years. After about six months or so, Dwight and I agreed that we wanted to be married. He said that he would start looking for a ring right away. I was elated and immediately called my parents, for I knew that they were really worried about my happiness. They were delighted because they knew this was a good man for me, you know how parents can tell.

I called my roadie and we started to prepare for the wedding. I felt like a young girl again. But my happiness wasn't to last for very long. One evening in September of 1993, I began to experience severe pain under my left arm. I had been feeling it for the last few days. I didn't think much of it then but now it made me stop and take notice. I reached under my arm and nothing was there but as I started to remove my hand it brushed across my left breast and I stopped breathing for a few minutes. Prior to that day I had never felt anything in my breast when showering.

When I could finally breathe again, my heart was racing and I was sweating profusely, it felt like my head was about to explode, and I cried out, oh GOD, please don't let this be what I think it is. I then proceeded to call my parents house and Dwight answered the phone. I shouted Dwight please help me, please God no, don't let this be happening. Dwight please come home I found a lump in my breast, it's very big. I'm screaming at the top of my voice, "it wasn't there before; where did it come from?" My husband was there in about five minutes. As he entered the house he hollered out "Phyllis where are you", barely audible, I said "I'm up here."

I was in a state of shock, as Dwight took the stairs, he was taking two steps at a time. When he finally got to me I was hysterically crying, he wrapped his arms around me and told me to calm down, he then said "let me see it." When I lifted my top he touched it, and I could see the look of terror in his frightened eyes, even though he tried to hide it. He was so upset that he said, "come on let's go to the emergency room", I said no, "I work at the clinic, they can check it out tomorrow." The rest of the night I couldn't sleep, so I spent the night talking to God, asking why me? Dwight held me close the remainder of the night. When I went to work in the morning I told my friend Bertie, who was a nurse at the clinic, she happened to be working with the surgeon, Dr. Robertson. She put me on his schedule, as a walk in, then I was told that I would be called when he was ready for me. I went back to work as usual as the medical record's clerk for the pediatric department. But I didn't get any work done as you can imagine. Later that morning she called me and proceeded to introduce me to the surgeon, I had seen him in the clinic a few times, but really didn't know him. He asked me what the problem was, and then I was told to lay on the table, as I lay there looking up to the heavens, I prayed, "Dear GOD please don't let it be cancer." He told me step by step what he was doing and what I would feel, A needle aspiration was done, which is a needle injection into the lump to see if fluid is drawn from it. Drawing fluid would mean a cyst. My deepest gut feeling was right, no fluid. I could see the sad look on both of their faces. Right then and there I knew I had breast cancer, the sweat was running all over me, before this I hardly got a cold. Dr. Robertson suggested a mammogram first and then a biopsy to follow, be ordered a mammogram done as soon as possible since I had never had one done before. I thought you didn't need one until late forties or fifty, I had just turned forty-two that year and I thought I had plenty of time. I now see why it is so important to get your baseline mammogram done and to be educated about at what age you should have it done. The thoughts that ran through my head in those weeks that followed were unreal. I didn't sleep, couldn't sleep because I was afraid I wouldn't wake up. Dr. Casselli had to give me a prescription for sleeping pills so I could get some rest, thoughts of death clouded my every waking moment, I had to sleep. In the next few days my mammogram was done, it was very, very, very nerve wrecking to have to sit and wait for the results, and to make matters worse the technician took the test twice. I sat there nervously twisting my fingers, and praying with all my heart and saying that this nightmare would be over soon. It felt like my heart was going to burst out of my chest, from the severe pounding. The technician came out with a female that she introduced to me as the radiologist. The doctor asked me when and how I found the lump? She then conveyed to me that the lump looked suspicious and that the result would be sent to my doctor, who would then order a biopsy. The rest of that day is really still a blur to me, for my life was about to take a drastic change. Dr. Robertson called after he received that report, it came back abnormal and we needed to get a biopsy done as soon as possible because of the size of the lump. Where did this thing come from and why wasn't it felt until now? This was a question I asked over and over again to myself.

Why was GOD doing this to me? The biopsy was done on October 5, 1993 at JOHN F KENNEDY MEMORIAL HOSPITAL, who I worked for. It was only a couple of weeks after finding the lump, everything was moving so fast since the discovery, which I now believe saved my life. Lying on the table the day of the biopsy, I remember saying, "0. K." GOD this is it, please, please let it be benign, you got my attention, you scared me into acknowledging your presence, and I promise I'll do better. The procedure was over and the doctor told me I would hear from him in about a week. You can't imagine what I went through those next few days, it was sheer terror, if this was truly cancer my life was over like so many other people I knew that died from this disease. In all of these years why had they not found a cure for this? Men walking on the moon but there is nothing to cure this thing? Dr. Robertson took very long to get back to me, so I thought, but my nerves were a wreck and I needed to know. Deep down inside maybe I didn't want to hear, because I already knew the answer. I called his office, he wasn't there and I was about to go crazy, so I called back a few hours later, he still wasn't available. The receptionist said she would have him call me as soon as he came in. That afternoon when the phone rang I almost couldn't answer, this was the call that would let me know if I would live or die, so I thought at the time. Softly, I said hello, on the other end was Dr Robertson, also speaking softly, he said, "Phyllis are you alone?" when I heard those words, the bedroom started to spin, my heart stopped beating, I couldn't breathe, Why didn't I wait for Dwight to come home before I called? I felt light headed and was about to pass out when I heard the doctor calling my name. He said "Phyllis are you alright?" Am I alright? I will never be alright again. Everything went black and I could see nothing, in my head I just kept saying, I'm going to die, I will never see my parents, sisters, my brother, Dwight, family, friends. At this time I knew nothing about chemotherapy. After what seemed like an eternity, I finally said to the doctor, "continue", he said, "Phyllis it's malignant", you have breast cancer. I just hung up the phone and started to scream, nothing was coming out, for a few seconds, I couldn't scream but my mouth was wide open. All I could think of was that I was forty-two and dying of a disease I really don't know anything about, this thing was growing inside of me and I never knew it was there. It was quietly trying to kill me and I couldn't do anything about it. Suddenly there they were, there they were. The Salem Light Cigarettes. I should have stopped smoking years ago like I said I would do. I grabbed the pack and started to rip each one apart, one by one saying, "you killed me, it's your fault." I had only heard death from cancer, associated with smoking. Not even thinking about grandmother, Nanny, who died from cancer, and she never smoked a day in her life.

After I could breathe again I picked up the phone and the first person I called was my oldest sister, Carol, I don't know why I didn't call my parents first. When

Carol answered I shouted "the doctor just called and I have cancer." There was silence for a few seconds before Carol could speak. You have to know that all my immediate family knew of cancer was that our grandparents both died of it. So I'm sure this crossed each of their minds, is my sister going to die? After it all sunk in we began to grab for our faith, we had to get over the initial shock. When she was able to speak she said, "calm down, calm down, are you alone?" I answered. "Yes", Dwight is at work but I'm on my way to mom's house, I have to get out of this house. By the time I got myself together and made it to my moms, she and Elaine were waiting for me. I entered the house crying, "please help me, I have cancer, I'm going to die, mom please help me, I don't want to die and leave you." My mother was holding me so very tight as if to say, you can't take my child if I hold onto her, and I felt the same way. If I was to die that very moment I was taking my mother so I wouldn't be alone. Elaine also held onto me and my mom, so the three of us were locked in an embrace, crying and not wanting to let go, for I didn't want to leave them so soon. When I could get myself together, I realized that I had to compose myself for my mom, she was crying so badly that she was moaning. "No Lord, No Lord, not my child, please don't take my child." Elaine sat me down and gave me some water, as I was sipping it, someone was coming in the door, it was my sister Carol and my two aunts, Louise and Reedie, they came as soon as they heard. My aunt Louise said we have to stop crying and pray like we have never prayed before. We all immediately started to a pray and ask the Lord for my healing. Afterward, the two aunts held me and said "we believe you are being healed as we speak, you must believe Phyllis" I was still in a daze but I shook my head yes. The rest of that day remains a blur, even until today. I returned to work the next day to see the doctor and get started on what needed to be done. Before I returned to work, Dwight came home, I gave him the bad news, but he always had the faith that I would be fine. He held me and I cried myself to sleep.

Dr. Robertson referred me to an Oncologist at another hospital that was very far from where I live. I objected, he then suggested that I see my primary doctor to get a referral for a hospital that was closer and I picked Graduate Hospital. This hospital is closer, only fifteen minutes away. Dr. Helene Casselli worked with me at the clinic, she was also my friend. The two of us would arrive at work before our shift because we enjoyed our jobs. We often talked in my office or hers about almost everything. This particular day, she first gave me the results of the mammogram and said, "Why does it always happen to the good ones?" She then shared with me that her mom, who was a crossing guard, like my oldest sister Carol, had passed away from breast cancer, but she said you will make it because of your strong will and your zest for life. I kept everyone at work laughing, my coworkers, Mary and Barbara would look for me to have lunch with them, so I could take their minds off the days stress, even if just for an hour. Dr. Casselli told me to call the American Cancer Society and tell them I was recently diagnosed with breast cancer and if they could recommend an Oncologist. I immediately called and they gave me Dr. Patricia Ford and I also asked them to send me some literature on breast cancer and chemotherapy and radiation. I selected a female doctor because I believed she would be more sensitive to my needs, and I was right, she is a superb Oncologist. I called and was given an October 15th appointment, the receptionist suggested that I have my records and all my x-rays sent to their office, so that when I come for my appointment with Dr. Ford she would have looked over everything. The day of the consultation she had read my records and told Dwight and I that she wanted me to see a Radiation Oncologist. She recommended Dr Nichini who was in the building. I made an appointment to see him on October 18, at which time he told me that he also had received my records and that he and Dr. Ford had decided on a course of treatment. My sisters Sharon and Cathy had attended this consultation with me because Dwight was unable to make it. I was elated that they went with me because I was still in a daze and could not remember everything told to me that day, except that I would get three months of chemo before the mastectomy and three months after the surgery, followed by seven weeks of Radiation, Monday through Friday. During my consultation with Dr. Ford was when I told the doctor that I was to be married in May of 1994 and I wanted to know if I could still plan to be married, she answered "I don't see why not". That is when I asked about a lumpectomy, which is the removal of the lump and some of the lymphnodes under the arm. This is done to spare taking the entire breast. I had read in the literature that was sent to me from the American Cancer Society, that more and more doctors were performing this type of surgery. But the doctor informed me that in my case the lump was too large and she felt that it would be in my best interest to remove the entire breast to be sure to get all of the cancer.

This is why she and Dr. Nichini had decided on the course of my treatment to be three months prior to surgery and three months after, followed by seven weeks of radiation.

With tears running down my face, so heavy that I couldn't see, I turned to Dwight and said, "what do you think" and he said, "do whatever you have to do to save your life so that you will be my wife for a very long long time." I am very content with the choice we made that day. But isn't it ironic that just when the Lord answered my prayers for a good caring man to enter my life, I was about to lose my breast and maybe my life, I thought to myself. But as I realize now, he was sent by GOD to be there for me and help get me through.

At that time I was so concerned about living long enough to marry this wonderful man. The emotions still well up in me even to this day, the tears are flowing as I write these words, because I know how much Dwight has meant in my life and how [fought to stay here and become Mrs. Dwight Alexander.

Prior to this day I had also gotten an x-ray of the chest and a bone scan done, this was done to be sure that the cancer had not spread to other parts of the body. Praise the Lord, it had not. Between the two tests I was at the clinic practically all day and I was physically and mentally drained.

In the next few days I was preparing myself for the start of my chemo treatment. One morning as I lay in my bed still praying for a miracle so I wouldn't have to loose my breast, the phone rang, I was thinking it was probably one of my family members calling to check on me. When I picked up the phone it was a call from the hospital where I had the biopsy done, the hospital I also worked for. The female voice on the other end went on to say that she was calling from the pathology department and wanted to speak to Ms. Wilson, I replied this is she, she proceeded to say that there had been a mix up in the pathology slides and the results that I had received were not mine. My heart stopped beating and my breath stopped, all for a second or so, this was the opposite of being told you had breast cancer. Finally when I could speak I said "say that again," when she did, I thought this is the miracle I had been praying for so hard. You can't imagine what my feelings were at that time, because I still can't express them myself. Once I got myself together I said to the technician on the other line, "thank God!!!!" She said she was sorry for the mix up, and I replied "this means that I don't have breast cancer?" She replied "that's right." At that time I never thought about the fact that the doctor didn't call me with such news. I was elated to hear those words that I didn't question it. After I hung up I said, "thank you Lord", over and over again with my hands up in the air holding them up to give him praise. I have to call my mother and all my family that were home, not excluding the others but they would be told later. When mom answered the phone I couldn't hold it anymore, I shouted out "mom I don't have cancer, they said it was a mistake and there was a mix up," and I'm crying and I praised the Lord. I was just rambling on, when mom finally said, "Phyllis slow down, mommy can't understand what your saying." When I could get breath I began to speak slowly now, because I was out of breath. Then I went on to tell her exactly what happened. She started to cry and shout out, "PRAISE THE LORD."

Then we both started to cry because we believed that GOD had performed HIS miracle.

I could not wait for Dwight to get home, he will be elated and we can now go on with our plans to be married. Later that day after I had called my brother, he was the only one I called at work, he was very happy for me. But you have got to know brother, he doesn't show much emotion because he says something always happens to us, meaning my immediate family, when we get too excited. He was right as usual. That evening as I was preparing a special dinner for Dwight to surprise him with the good news the phone rang, I never thought it would be anybody other than family members calling after they heard the good news. Rut when I answered the phone, I knew something was wrong, because the voice was that of a white female who started the conversation with "Ms. Wilson, I am sorry to tell you that there wasn't a mistake, we found that your slide was the one that verifies that you do have breast cancer." Was this really happening? What is going on? God why are you doing this to me all over again? I didn't realize at the time that he was really testing my faith, that he would truly cure me of cancer, for good. I asked, after I could breath again, "how could this happen?" She replied, "there is a Phyllis Wilson and a Patricia Wilson and for some reason the two first names were mixed up." I said, "are you people able to read?" Did you all graduate from school? I was trying to hurt someone because I was hurting so bad. I just hung up and sat down and stared at the wall for what seemed like hours. When I got myself together, I called my mother to tell her the bad news, she answered the phone and when I said hello, she said "hi baby" with such happiness in her voice for she believed that her child didn't have cancer. How was I going to break it to her that I did have cancer. I just came out and told her what had just happened. She knew I was very upset so she hid her emotions for me. All she could get out was, "oh baby I'm so sorry mommy is so sorry." I'll talk to you later mom, is all I could get out, and then I just hung up and before I knew it the tears were flowing, I kept thinking about how it felt for that short time, being cancer free. My Dwight never got to see the joy I felt for that brief time.

Once I calmed myself down I called my brother back and when he answered the phone I said "you were right again BOO, nothing ever works out for us that is good." To that he replied "what happened, what's the matter, what is wrong?" "I still have cancer Boo," tears running, "they said it was a mistake after all, they had two Wilsons, one Phyllis and one Patricia," he said "how can they get Phyllis and Patricia mixed up?" In a daze I replied, "I asked them that also." He said, "I'm so sorry sis, I didn't want to be right about something like this." I then started to ball like I'm doing now because the incident is so vivid in my mind. He said,

"I will take care of this, someone will pay for this." My brother is the Business Manager for Local 427 of the Sanitation workers of the City of Philadelphia. When he speaks people listen. My brother worked his way up from trash man, throwing trash, to the position he holds today, no one gave him anything, he worked for everything he has. I truly respect my big brother and I often said, before meeting Dwight that I wanted to marry a man just like my brother and father, and I did. His word is bond, because later that night I received another call from the hospital from the director, Mr. Holmes who expressed his sincere apology for the incident. I knew he meant well but that didn't erase the fact that my life was again traumatized. People told me that I could sue, but then I was concerned about getting over this so that I could again begin to prepare myself for the days ahead. But when I think about it now, those involved really got away with just a slap on the hand.

On October 22, 1993 as Dwight and I sat in Dr. Ford's office that fateful day I thought to myself, here we go DEAR LORD, in my journal I had written about how terrified I really was, but wanted to stay strong for Dwight, for he was also going through some rough times. As we proceeded to the chemo suites, my stomach was doing flops. Inside the site there were chairs made of leather lined up in a straight line. People were sitting in them all hooked up to IV poles, and as I passed each one, down to the very end of the line, they all looked up to me with such compassion, for they all had been in my shoes before. Each of them had to go through that first time.

The nurse was so very kind and gentle in her speaking and in helping me through this traumatic time. As she inserted the IV into my hand she explained everything along the way.

The combination of medication that was given to me is called, 5FU, and I asked which one makes my hair come out and she replied, the ADRIAMYCIN. Are you ready she asked? As ready as I can get, as the medication was pushed into my veins she warned that I would feel very warm, I held onto Dwight's hand and I was praying that I would not break it. Warm was an understatement it felt as if my veins were about to explode. GOD help me, it burns so bad, I thought to myself as I bit into my lip. The treatment lasted an hour and the nurse stayed with me the entire time. I was given crackers and juice prior to the administration of the medication and it felt as If I was going to bring it up. I told the nurse and she immediately called for another nurse to bring me a emesis basin. Fortunately I didn't vomit, I was afraid to put my body through any more than what it was already experiencing.

After the treatment was completed, I looked around the room and everyone was staring at me with a look of sheer exhilaration. For I had also gotten through my first chemotherapy treatment. The nurse then gave me my instruction sheet that stated what I should eat and what I should do for the rest of the day. which included plenty of rest, she did not have to tell me that because I extremely tired, the treatment had zapped all of my strength. I was also told that a port, which is a device implanted under the skin above my right breast, would have to be put in as soon as possible. She continued to say that the remaining treatments would be given through this because the medication would, blow out my veins, which it did. And they could also draw blood from this, which made it much easier, and I thank GOD for it.

What got me though that first treatment was saying over and over "THE LORD GOD WILL NOT FAIL YOU OR FORSAKE YOU." My faith grew stronger and stronger and HE continues to Guide me through all of my trials and tribulations and even though I'm not able to work, I do miss working. He is keeping me busy by writing this book to help others. My chemo treatments were scheduled for two Fridays on and two Fridays off, this would give my good cells time to heal.

On October 24, 1993, a couple of days later, I started to experience some of those side effects I was told about, aside from the usual nausea, I was feeling stomach burning that I would imagine was equal to drinking acid, later those side effects grew to include mouth sores, rashes, and a variety of others that you will read about later, I called the doctor's answering service because it was in the evening when I first started to have these symptoms.

She said they were indeed the side effects she had spoken of and immediately called in a prescription for medication that would ease the symptoms. During this time I was still praying for a miracle to save my breast but I also prayed, GOD, YOUR WILL BE DONE.

The port insertion was scheduled for October 28, 1993, it was to be done by Dr. Robertson, I was very concerned because the next day I was to receive chemo treatment and I didn't want the site to be too sore for the injection, then I would have to worry about the soreness and the nausea. Before I knew it, the day was upon me to get the port inserted, sometimes it made my head whirl for this was moving so fast. We arrived early because I had to get a chest x-ray and cardiogram done. I got all checked in and was taken up to my room. The technician was called, and my test were done at bedside, as she took the paper out of the machine she turned and looked at me and asked if I had ever had heart problems and I answered no, than I asked her why did she ask that, Dwight and I looked at each other as if to say what now. She replied because you have an irregular heartbeat. I told her that I had never had any problems before receiving chemo. The nurse was called and told to call Dr. Robertson and the cardiologist. By now my nerves were shot, and I could not take anymore bad news, but I also knew that GOD doesn't put on you anymore than you can bear. I was always told that I'm a very strong woman and my mom said that even as a little girl, I was told by my grandfather, her father, that I would grow up to be a tough cookie and I did, God rest his soul. Many thoughts ran across my mind as we waited for the doctors to come. Dwight saw the look on my face and rubbed my hand and said "hang in there you're doing good." Just then the cardiologist along with Dr. Robertson came into my room, the doctor took a look at the results, the cardiologist spoke first, "you have a heart murmur, did you know that?" I answered no, I didn't. This was not told to my mother when I was born, she was only told that I would have flat feet, that's all. He went on to say that he would suggest that the surgery be cancelled because he didn't know if it was a good idea for me to be put to sleep. Dr. Robertson checked the results and he agreed. I said, listen doctors, "I finally, got my nerves together and now you tell me my surgery has to be cancelled." Before I could go on Dwight spoke up and asked what else could be done to continue with the procedure? Both doctors said it could be done under local anesthesia, which means, instead of going to sleep I would be injected in the area where the port would be inserted with a numbing medication so I would not feel the surgery. I said, let's do it, and we proceecied to the operating room. Once inside the room I was told that after the injection, If I felt anything to let them know immediately, they didn't have to tell me that. The surgery began, and I lay there looking up to the heavens and talking to the good LORD, as the doctors did their thing. The procedure was to last about forty-five minutes but half way through I actually felt the knife cutting into my flesh and I screamed out, "I feel the cutting, stop until you give me more medication," The doctor answered, O.K. Phyllis you'll feel better in a few seconds. Which I did and the rest Of the surgery was uneventful. I went back to my room to rest for awhile and to have some snacks because I was told not to eat anything or drink anything after ten o'clock, p.m. After they watched me for a few hours I was discharged and went home to sleep, for in the last few days leading up to this, I didn't sleep well at all. Later that night I was in excruciating pain, even with the pain medication. I couldn't sleep, Dwight was sleeping so good, he needed the rest and I didn't want to wake him. So I went into another room and called my sister, Sharon. When she answered the phone I said, "sorry for calling you so late but I can't sleep and I need to talk to someone." She said it's alright, and as we started to speak the tears started coming. I shared with her how I was so very scared, and that even knowing what GOD had already done for me, the human side of me, was still hoping that I would make it. I was now crying out loud and she was saying "Phyllis you will be fine, just keep holding onto your faith" to that I replied, I'm trying so hard sis, because I don't want to die and leave you all, but now Sharon was also crying very hard and that's when Dwight entered the room and took the phone, and spoke into it saying to both of us, no one is going to die and now both of you try and get some rest.

Because of the port insertion my chemo treatment the next day went very smoothly, When I mentioned to the nurse that I did have the port, but the area was so sore, she proceeded to inject into the area very gently. This was so much better than putting it through my veins.

After each of my chemo treatments were done, I would make a dash for my parent's house where I felt safe and cared for. Dwight was working and I couldn't stand the idea of being alone, during this time. There my parents would take turns giving me soup, because this a the only thing I could hold down, after receiving chemo. More and more side effects started to show their ugly faces as treatments continued. Added to the few I mentioned earlier stomach burning and mouth sores, there were now several others like cramping in my stomach, cramping in my legs, throat closing, tightness in the chest, severe bone pain in the chest area and severe shortness of breath which I swear has to do with my chronic asthma and respiratory problems. Also, my period stopped, which wasn't a bad thing, and I was always constipated, most all of these conditions still persist today, but compared to what i've been through, I can deal with them. It's only by the grace of GOD, that I'm alive and able to be here to share my blessings, by spreading the word that you too can be a survivor.

As I sat on my couch saying my morning prayers this day, November 4, 1993, I had such a spiritual experience that I found myself dropped to my knees. During the prayers I said aloud, "LORD I KNOW YOU ARE HEALING ME, BUT LORD COULD YOU PLEASE GIVE YOUR CHILD A SIGN?" After only a few minutes, my left pinky finger started to tremble uncontrollably and I felt a kind of sensation go up my left arm, to my chest area where the cancer was discovered by me. Now on my knees, I shouted "PRAISE YOU LORD, PRAISE YOUR NAME, THANK YOU DEAR LORD, I couldn't stop Praising and Thanking Him enough for he had answered my plea for a sign. I knew that November day that I was truly healed, I just had to go through the mastectomy, but I was definitely going to live. The incident only lasted for a few minutes but that feeling of great peace and love lasted sometime. As I write these words I can still remember that heavenly feeling. And again I am choked up with emotion. I had to share this very spiritual event with my mother so I called her, right away. When she answered the phone I said, "mom the HOLY SPIRIT has just filled me with this feeling of GOD's unconditional love, and then I went on to share with her what had just happened.

My mom was raised Baptist, but when she married my father who is Catholic, as is his brothers and sisters, she took religious instructions and became Catholic, now she is the most dedicated person in our family to our religion.

GOD had showed me that I would be around for Christmas and all the rest of the holidays for years to come. I also realized that I would be here to become Mrs. Dwight Alexander. GOD is good, all the time.

The next day I went out to look for a wig, I felt so very happy to know that I was going to make it, that I no longer worried about my hair loss. I just had to remain strong, to get through these trials and tribulations, I knew I could do that. Looking for a wig wasn't so bad, now that I had my answer, I looked at several wigs before I found the one that was waiting for me. As I passed by the window, there it sat, my wig, just waiting for me. It was the exact color that I had my own hair streaked, it was also the way I styled my hair for years. I thought to myself this is eerie, then I realized it was the LORD at work again. I entered the store and as the sales person approached me I told her I would like to see that, pointing to the wig in the window. When she returned with it in her hand she looked at the wig and then at my own hair, she looked up again and before she could say anything, I said, I know it looks exactly like my hair. She then asked if I wanted to try it on. I really didn't have to, for I knew It would be perfect. But I did and I was absolutely right. I purchased it, in the nick of time because my hair started to come out several days later. Another nightmare began to unfold November 9, 1993. As Dwight and I prepared for bed that night I had taken my shower first and was now talking to him, he was now in the shower. While combing my hair I noticed excessive amounts of hair in the comb. I had fooled myself into thinking maybe mine would be the exception and not come out, even though my Roadie had warned me that just as hers had fallen out, I'd better prepare myself for hair loss, because I don't know of anyone who didn't lose all of their hair, or almost all of it. Within a week I lost more and more and shortly there after, I noticed I had bald spots. The night I noticed the bald spots I broke down and cried hysterically, it was devastating. And for all of you who tried to comfort me, which I appreciate, by telling me it will grow back, you have to understand that it's not what you need to hear at that moment, because you stand before me with a head full of hair, so my Roadie was the only one who had the experience to say those words. My hair was always thick, not all that long, but a nice length. It wasn't just the hair, as any survivor can tell you, it's about all of the emotions you go through during this traumatic time. On this particular night as I was crying, Dwight came into the bedroom and gave me a hug, It will be alright Phyllis. He then disappeared into another room, he could never stand to see me cry. When he returned, he called out my name and said, Look Phil, and I looked up, there he stood, my wig on his head just sitting on top, plus it was backward. My husband is six foot six and very slender, picture it, We laughed so hard, and when we finally got up off the floor, I felt so much better.

On one of my Roadie, Elaine's many visits, I shared with her about my hair lose, and she suggested that I let her cut what was left of my hair down, so it won't look so traumatic as it continues to come out. She was a licensed hair stylist and was doing my hair prior to this ordeal. We often bring up how no one trusted her to do their hair right after graduating from school. One saturday afternoon as we sat in her house we were talking about hair styles and the jerri curl was mentioned, it was a new curly perm. I asked Elaine could she do a curl she said "I could sure try.' Her sisters said, "not on my hair" I felt so bad for her, your own blood don't trust you, I thought to myself. She is just like a sister to me, because she understands me more than anyone, and accepts me for who I am even when I have one of my mood swings. So I spoke up and said, Roadie, I trust you, you can give me a jerri curl and she did a beautiful job. Then her sisters saw how nice mine looked and they wanted theirs done also, we said we would never forget that day, and we haven't.

So she did cut my hair down to a very short style and it didn't look bad at all, in fact I grew to like the haircut very much. Elaine shared with me recently, that the day she cut my hair it was very emotional for her also. She brought back to my attention how she kept disappearing into my kitchen, she said as she was cutting my hair, her eyes kept tearing up and she pretended to be laughing it up, with my husband in the kitchen, but she was getting herself together. She went on to say that she couldn't believe that her Roadie was going through the same experience years later, that she herself had been through years earlier. She stated, It was very hard for her to have to be doing this all over again, and this time for her best friend. We both filled up over the phone, as we reminisced about our bouts with the disease. She didn't have breast cancer, but she had cancer just the same. After Elaine's initial cut, Dwight kept up the maintenance on my hair, until it eventually was all gone.

The days that followed, I started to wear the hats that sisters Sharon and Cathy had purchased for me. On the days when I did wear the wig, I would keep a scarf handy, at my parent's and at my house in case I wanted to take off the hot wig. I only felt comfortable to sit bald headed around my immediate family. During this time I was experiencing severe hot flashes, which my brother Boo teased me about all the time. He would say it was from my age not the medication my period had stopped and I was going through menopausal symptoms, combined with the Tamoxifen, which is a anti-cancer pill, with side effects such as water retention, weight gain and hot flashes so it was a double bubble. They have calmed down a great deal now that I have been taking the medication for two years soon to be three, Praise the LORD. But I must have gained about thirty pounds in that time. I'm fat, but I'm alive and my husband loves me regardless of the weight. A slender person I wasn't but I watched my weight all the time and remained a size thirteen/fourteen until my diagnosis, I have my friends laughing when I tell them I must have been born that size because, I've never been that much smaller even as a child, so I was content being my size, for I knew I would never be a model. At fourteen, I was that size in my oldest sister's wedding.

During one of my chemo treatments, as I sat with the medication entering my body, I wondered why the Lord was sparing my life. This answered my question: On the job one of those rare days, when I was feeling pretty good my phone rang in my office, at the other end was Bill, a Physician's Assistant, who worked in the walk-in section of the clinic. He asked if I would like to speak to a woman just diagnosed with breast cancer. I replied, 'sure I'll do what I can." Shortly thereafter there was a knock on my door, before I could say come in I asked the Lord to give me the words to comfort this lady, as she entered I turned to see a distraught person with the same fear in her face that I had in mine that dreadful day back in September. We immediately embraced as if we had known each other for years. The two of us cried as I whispered in her ear, I know, I know, I was patting her back and she was patting mine. Then I spoke, "make up your mind as I did, to fight for your life don't let cancer win, we are in control of our bodies and we have to show it." I told her of my recently being told that I also have breast cancer and that I would have to have a mastectomy, which didn't mean she would too. After talking for a while, she calmed down and said, she didn't know how she was going to make it home if I hadn't been there for her. I knew at that moment when she said that, I had made a difference in someone's life, this was my purpose for being on this earth. The Lord had showed me what I asked of HIM several times before. All these years and my mission was finally revealed to me that day. Her name is Yvonne Barnes and she is doing fine and she only had to have a lumpectomy done, with chemo She's doing great. She kept in contact with me after that, and she still comes to holler at me whenever she comes to the clinic. A few months before I went out for a leave of absence another lady was sent to me who was also very upset, when she came to the clinic she was in the lab and was telling the tech, Janet, that she had been diagnosed with breast cancer and started to cry. Janet called me to see if it was alright for her to send the lady back to my office, I said, certainly, I'll do what I can. This lady was also choked up, you can imagine. I held her as she began to sob and told her that if she believed in GOD she had better be talking to him and asking him to spare her life. We kept in contact for a while and then I lost her phone number and I have been praying that she would call me so I can see how she's doing. But since she hasn't called me maybe she lost my number. So I pray she is doing fine. Now I see that if I wasn't there for both those ladies, when they needed someone who had been through it, they may not have had the courage to fight for their very lives, so I feel very blessed to have been there for each of them.

It was now the holidays and on my job we were preparing for our annual Christmas party, which my sisters and I look forward to every year.

In the meantime I went to see Dr. Seinge, who was recommended by Dr. Ford and who would be doing the surgery, on December 20, 1993. She was a very gentle person, who spoke with a beautiful accent as she went on to explain what she would be doing and since I had decided to get reconstruction surgery, she explained that once she was done with the mastectomy, Dr. Montiero who I had also recently seen, would take over and put in the expander, that he would inject with saline weekly to stretch my skin. After the skin was sufficiently stretched he then would put in the permanent implant, Saline implant.

Since our Christmas Party was scheduled for December 18, 1993, two days before my surgery, I planned to have myself a complete ball which I did. My sisters and their husbands or boyfriends, Elaine and her boyfriend Leon and Dwight and I. We did the electric slide, and we had the floor, because my sisters and I know about four different versions of the line dance. People still talk about how Phyllis and her family stole the party.

The night before the surgery, Dwight and I talked and I shared with him how I felt about this being the last night, that I would have two breast. I also asked him how he felt about his soon to be bride coming into the marriage ill-formed. His reply was "Phyllis I will tell you again I Love you, not just your breast, I Love you for who you are and what you have meant to my life. You are the best thing that has happened to my life." We embraced with tears in our eyes, he then said to me now go to sleep you need to get some rest. Gee, I said to myself, this is what they say Love really feels like, I truly love this man.

On the morning of December 20, 1993, I wrote this in my journal: This is the day my breast will be removed because of breast cancer, but I will live, I'm just a little down, but I'm only human. That day is vivid in my mind, my mother and all my sisters and my Dwight, all went to the hospital to be with me, my brother and dad couldn't make it. But I believe they couldn't take it, the two of them are very strong men but when it comes to their family they just can't stand to see us in pain and feeling so helpless. So I really did understand. My brother Boo, as we call him, and I fought all the time as children, not fist fight, just arguing, and since we have grown into adults we are very very close and it was just too painful for them. As we sat in the surgical lounge, Dwight tried to make us laugh, usually we do, but this day we could only smile. My heart went out to my sister Carol because she was so very upset, I could see it in her eyes as she sat across from me, so even though I was petrified, I tried to hold up for all of them. I knew if I broke down they would all lose it, but the harder I tried the harder it became, to keep the tears away. Looking from one to the other, the human side took over again and I prayed to the LORD to please let me see them all again and my inner self knew that I would. When I was finally called, I reach up and gave Dwight a kiss and said see you later. I then waved to my mother and sister, for I knew if I hugged them I might never let go and maybe even change my mind about the surgery. And

I knew this had to be done to save my life. Here comes the tears again. Dwight reached down and hugged me and as I walked away from his embrace, I never turned back around. I couldn't stand to see their faces, and I knew it wasn't possible, but I wanted to holler "Dwight please come with me, don't make me go alone." Deep down inside I knew I wasn't alone, GOD was there with me and my loved ones, all of them who passed away and last but not least, my guardian angel was hand in hand walking with me.

As the nurse was preparing me for the surgery, I recognized another nurse, who use to work with me at St, Agnes hospital in the operating room. I was the instrument technician there for fourteen years, so I was very familiar with the medical terminology and of course all the instruments they were going to use.

The IV line was put in and we then waited a few minutes for my surgeons to come in an say hello before I went to sleep. After speaking with them, I was told to count back from one hundred. As I started to count I remember feeling very drowsy and only got to ninety seven. I then awoke to the sound of a nurse calling my name, she said wake up Ms. Wilson, which was my name, from a first marriage. She went on to say that my surgery went very, very, well and that I was now in the recovery room. The first thing I said was that I was very cold and I was shaking, she then brought me another blanket and asked me if that felt better, which it did. I then asked, if they had took the breast she said they did and the doctor would talk to me when I got back to my room. Where's Dwight, I want to see him and my family. She replied you can see them back at your room. Then I said to myself I forgot to thank GOD and then I went on to say DEAR GOD, THANK YOU SO VERY MUCH. After awhile, I was taken back to my room, but I was in and out of sleep and don't remember much after that, except that I was wheeled into the room, I did see my mother and sisters and then I closed my eyes again and this time when I opened them there he stood my man, the tears started to pour from our eyes as he leaned down to kiss me. I spoke softly in his ear, "Hi Boop" a nickname I gave him, "I made it." Then I hear my mother step up, I looked up and said, "Hi Mommy", I sounded like a child and I felt like a child who missed their mommy, she held my hand and leaned over to kiss my cheek. As she did the tears from her eyes were falling on my face. She said "mommy is here baby, mommy is here." I didn't ever want to let her hand go again, and as I was drifting back off to sleep, I could hear my sisters crying, but I knew it was alright to sleep now.

When I opened my eyes again, hours later I felt pain, body ripping pain, that hurt throughout my entire body. I cried out for Dwight, the pain, help me, the pain. One of my sisters ran out of the room to find a nurse to get some pain medication. The anesthesia must have worn off I thought to myself. The nurse arrived and gave me the medication and said that I would be feeling better soon. As the medicine was taking effect my surgeon entered the room, she informed me that I did very well and that she had gotten all the cancer. She went on to inform me that of thirty lymph nodes taken from my arm, only three were cancerous, which is good. And once I resume my chemotherapy and completed my radiation treatment, I would be fine. One of my sisters asked the doctor what are my chances for a complete recovery. She answered, very, very good. I now spoke up and asked what percentage of complete recovery will I have? She smiled and said, "Phyllis I would say your percentage of complete recovery would be about 90%." When I heard that I was elated, GOD had truly healed me. The cancer was gone from my body, it meant losing my breast, but I was going to live, PRAISE THE LORD. Later that day after my family had left and I was in and out of sleep I vaguely remember this lady entered the room and she asked if I was Phyllis Wilson? I answered, yes I am, she proceeded to tell me that she was from a program to help women who had Breast Cancer. As she spoke I started to wince in pain and she said, I see you are in a lot of pain, I will come back later, I must have went off to sleep again because that's all I remember, I never saw her leave. This just came back to me for when I called years later to join the program I was asked if there was a volunteer from the REACH TO RECOVERY program that came to see me, and I answered no, because I truly didn't remember.

The nurses were extremely caring and gentle people. This was important to me, because I was very scared and very very sore. They all went out of their way to see that I was comfortable.

Whenever the doctors came to visit me, they informed me that I was doing very good and if I continued to do well, I would be able to go home, it sounded so good to hear those words. Christmas was in a few days and I wanted to be home for this special special holiday, so I made sure to do exactly as I was told. The doctor said, if I could start to urinate without the foley, that would be a good sign that I could go home, and also the other problem would be the drains. Anything that I needed to do I was willing for I knew that would get me home that much quicker. The nurses on that surgical floor were exceptional people and went beyond their call of duty. This is still fresh in my mind today.

The next couple of days are taken right from my journal that I kept, I would like to share my feelings with you all.

December 23, 1993, THANK GOD, I made it, and I PRAISE HIS NAME! I'm being discharged today, Sharon came to get me because I can't get in touch with Dwight fast enough. She will be here to get me around ten o'clock. I was very happy to see her and very happy to be going home in time for the holidays. First the doctors were to send me home tomorrow but GOD sent me home a day early.

December 24, 1993, GOD, I made it to Christmas Eve, so happy to be alive. Stayed with dad all day and am going to church with mom and Cathy. I'm going to Thank and PRAISE HIM for this miracle of life. Then went to Carol's house for her annual Christmas Eve party. Arm aching and swollen, started early this morning, was told to keep it propped up, and to be careful for lymphedema, which is fluid backed up in the arm that the nodes were removed from.

In church, as the priest was saying the Mass, 'I became so overwhelmed with emotion I began to sob. I was allowed to live, and now, was sitting in the LORD's house with my family and as I looked over my mom and sister were also choked up, our tears were tears of joy.

The following was written in my book in very large print.

DECEMER 25, 1993;

I MADE IT, PRAISE THE LORD, IT'S
CHRISTMAS DAY, I LOVE LIFE, I LOVE MY
FAMILY AND I LOVE MY FRIENDS, ELAINE
AND LEON, THEY ARE SPECIAL FRIENDS.
GOING TO DINNER AT MY PARENTS WITH
ALL MY FAMILY. I WASN'T SAD ABOUT NOT
HAVING CHILDREN THIS YEAR, I WAS
JUST SO GLAD TO BE ALIVE, I MADE IT.

The day after Christmas was spent at my brother's
house, we had a wonderful time. I couldn't have made
it without them all. These thoughts went through my
head, as I looked around my brothers house, because
there was such happiness. Everyone was celebrating
life for it could have easily been one of them coming
so close to dying.

One of the conditions, that allowed me to come home
early was that I would go home with a drain, that was
inserted into my side with a rubber tube, connected
to a device that looked much like a hand grenade. A
nurse was sent out for a few days to help me empty
it and to take my vital signs. But after only one day I
told her she didn't need to come again, because my
husband would take over once I showed him what
to do. When he came home that day I showed him
what needed to be done, and he immediately took
over, like I knew he would. What a man I have.

The next couple of weeks there was stiffness and pulling in my chest area. I had many, many days of severe pain that followed, but GOD brought me through them all. Those nights were the worse because I couldn't lie flat on my back and I sure couldn't lay on my side. Most nights I just lay awake asking GOD to please take away the pain, so that I could sleep. A good nights sleep was so very rare. The pain got so bad that I needed sleeping pills to get some rest, also I didn't want Dwight to be up with me all night. On my next visit to the surgeon she suggested arm exercises to loosen the chest muscles and make me more comfortable.

On January 10, 1994, I saw my cosmetic surgeon who also operated on me that day, he put in a implant called an expander. His name is Dr. Montiero and he was also very caring and very pleasant. We both were planning to be married soon and often discussed our plans, he was married a few months after me. He said that he would start to fill the expander with saline each week, once a week until my skin was stretched to accommodate my permanent implant. He said he would try to get it as close to the size of my right breast as possible.

This next day was taken from my journal, only another cancer survivor can identify with the following statement which came from my heart.

I really dread today, because I start chemo again today, I stopped my last round of chemo in December, right before my surgery. I LOVE JESUS, BUT THE TREATMENT IS SO ROUGH AND IT MAKES ME SO SICK I'M GRATEFUL THAT I'M ALIVE AND THAT THE CHEMO IS PART OF THE REASON, BUT IT'S LIKE I'M STARTING ALL OVER AGAIN. THE STOMACH BURNING, THE MOUTH SORES, CAN'T SWALLOW. THROAT CLOSING. LORD BLESS ME, LORD HELP ME!!!

The next day was my treatment and I was really depressed and I tried not to show it, but the staff knew me to well. All of the nurses stopped and patted me on the shoulder and said for me to hang in there. They saw that something was wrong right away, because usually I was so talkative, but not this day. Just when my stomach would start to feel better from the previous treatment, it was time for another. This went on for a total of six months. February was spent between chemo and going to Dr. Montiero, to have my expander filled, which entaled him inserting the tip of a syringe into skin which, then went inside of the expander.

Valentine day that year fell on chemo day, so when I finished treatment that day, I went home instead of going to my parent's house. I want to start to prepare a very special dinner for that wonderful man of mine. I didn't want to go out for dinner, I wanted it to be a cozy dinner for just the two of us, We had steak, baked potato and salad, it was a very nice evening, with candles also.

February 23, 1 994 (I was home in bed when Dwight came home shouting up the stairs for me. I answered, "here I am up here," which took a lot of effort because this particular treatment had really washed me out and I could hardly sit up. He came up the stairs two at a time. When he got to the bedroom, he asked how I felt and I told him this was one of bad days, my chest was hurting so much, from being so tight from the expander stretching my skin. I also told him that I was very, very queasy today, I just felt plain old rotten. He said I have something to make you feel better. He went on to get down on one knee, and pulled this velvet case of his pocket. He gave it to me and said open it, my hands were shaking when I opened it, I had never seen anything so beautiful in my entire life. It was sparkling so bright, he then took the ring from it's case and put it on my finger. I tried to sit up, but I was too weak, but I did manage to roll over. All I could say was, "oh Boop, it's beautiful." With tears in his eyes he said "Phyllis will you Marry me?" Tears were rolling down my face as I answered "oh yes, yes". This makes it official, it can't be official without a ring, he had been saving since the previous year. I could not stop looking at it. I did not want to take my eyes off of it. Dwight was right, when he said that it would make feel better, I didn't think about the pain for the rest of the night. I said to him, I feel like a million dollars. He replied, that's about how much it costs, but of course, it didn't, months later when I was given the paper to put away and saw how much it actually cost, I laughed and said, you were right, it is like a million dollars to us. Later that night as he lay sleeping, I said, "Lord you sent him into my life right on time" as the prayer says he doesn't always come when you call him but he's right on time, so very true. For here I lay bald headed, one breast, dark circles under my eyes and he still loved me enough, to want me to be his Wife. He's now my husband, my lover, my friend, and besides my Lord and Savior, he's the man. Words cannot express what I felt for this man. The closest that I can come to it, is to say I will be eternally grateful and will love him forever and ever.

I was married before and that marriage could never compare to this sincere love that this man feels for me. You can really tell when you are loved, when a man or woman stays with you through a dreaded disease, like cancer. I never imagined in my wildest dreams that a man could love me that much, but he does. I pray that all of you who have been diagnosed, and those of you who will be, that you have someone like my husband who will see you through.

By April I was getting very excited for soon it would be all over. I would get my strength back and my hair would have grown in enough for my wedding.

Since the diagnosis, I have thanked GOD for each and every day, and every birthday is like a holiday to me, because like many of us, I took life for granted.

I began to take therapy which was suggested to my doctors, to gain full use of my left arm. There was a time when I couldn't lift my arm at all, I just kept it close to my side, not moving it up or down. This made it very stiff and very sore. So I was referred to a BREAST CANCER PHYSICAL THERAPIST. The therapist assured me, that I would have back full use of am. At that time it was hard to believe, but GOD, it is back to normal. It took about a month, and she did a wonderful job, and she was an excellent people person, also. Thanks Linda. I was waiting to be called, I was given paper work to complete, as I gazed around the room, looking at the different machines, my eyes came upon a picture, I will never forget. My mouth dropped open, and I was amazed at what was on the wall before me. It was a drawing of a woman, standing with nothing on, from the waist up, I couldn't believe my eyes, there she stood with one breast, it literally took my breathe away. I had never seen anyone with one breast openly exposed like that. When my bandages were taken off in the hospital after the removal of the implant, I didn't look at myself, my husband looked for me. I didn't look for a very long time until he kept telling me it wasn't that bad, and he was right. Remember I had reconstructive surgery, which was done immediately after the mastectomy, so up until now, I had never seen anyone exposed like that, and for a long period of time, my husband didn't see me exposed either. The therapist was correct, I did regain full use of my arm, it still remains stiff sometime, but once I start to work it, it loosens up just fine.

April 22, 1994, that day will live in my memory forever, as my last day of chemotherapy. PRAISE THE LORD iii!!!! I remember sitting in the chair thinking to myself, this is my last day to have to go through this. I made it DEAR LORD, with your help. I told the staff that they were not getting rid of me so easily, I told them, I will be back for my check ups every one or two months. So this wasn't good-bye. They are like family to me and it remains that way today. THANK GOD, I now go every six months.

Now it was time to really get busy with my wedding plans, Elaine and I started to finish up the things we had begun. MY sister Sharon took me out to look for a dress, I had an idea of what I wanted to wear. The medication I was taking made me put on a lot of weight, and I needed to find something that would help hide some of the fat. We went to a few stores, before she suggested the one I purchased my dress from. I was excited as I went about getting things together. I quickly called Elaine, to see if she had gotten her dress yet, because she had been looking all along. She couldn't find anything she liked so the two of us went out one day and we agreed we would not stop until we got her dress. Which we did, after store, after store, after store. I didn't mind because I felt fine those days, after chemo was done, my hair started to grow back, it came in very fine, like baby hair, I loved it.

We had a small, but beautiful wedding, with Elaine, as maid of honor and Leon, her boyfriend as Dwight's best man, these were our best friends, the four of us spent a lot of time together. The morning of the wedding was like nothing I can explain, all of my prayers had been answered, and today, May 21, 1994, I was to become Mrs. Dwight Alexander. On this day, we would become man and wife, I liked the sound of those words. Today I would celebrate my life, and my future with my husband and friends and family. Just before we got ready to go to the community center, where we were married, my godson Vaughn, my brother-in-law and his wife and daughter all came to help us get ready. As Terry, my sister-in-law, called up to see if I was almost finished, I was shaking so bad I couldn't get my earrings in, but I finally did.

I was wearing a white dress with short sleeves, with matching swing coat. The dress was down to my knees, and the jacket was three quarters. There was gold beads on the collar and around the sleeves, with one big button at the top of the coat, that was gold also, with a large white pearl inside of it. My hat was also white, I guess you could call it a pill box hat, it had a short veil over it and it had gold buttons on it, I wore white satin pumps, with gold and pearl clips attached to the front, and I wore white sheer stockings with gold running down the side of them. If I must say so myself, I was beautiful. My skin had gotten darker from the chemo, and that white and gold up against my dark skin really set it off. My bouquet was made up of carnations, which were sprayed with gold, they were gorgeous.

Dwight was so very handsome, he wore a grey pin striped suite, with a beautiful blue shirt, and matching tie and handkerchief, that had a deeper shade of blue than the shirt. He dressed downstairs and I dressed upstairs, when I finally came down the stairs everyone said Phyllis you look so beautiful, and I felt better than I did before I was ill. When I started to see my man coming from the kitchen, we both filled up, for we had come a long way together. He was so handsome, I could hardly take my eyes off of him, As I thought to myself, I'm glad he belongs to me,.,

Elaine wore a suit that was very nice also, it was a beautiful color of blue, with a lovely pair of gold shoes and bag to match. When she came to my house that day I said "go Roadie".

Leon wore a grey suit also but it was a shade darker, he dresses nicely all of the time. We could not have picked better people, to share our special day by being in our wedding.

Our guest list had grown enormously, because my husband kept inviting everyone he came in contact with. Different people in the neighborhood, would come up to me and say I saw Dwight and he said I could come to the wedding. I told him to stop inviting people because we only had room for about one hundred guest. My family always did the cooking for all of my relatives weddings, you would think it was catered when we finished with the preparations. The day of the wedding there must have been close to one hundred and fifty, courtesy of Dwight. My sisters said, not to worry we always have more than enough food and liquor, and we did. The day after the wedding my sisters and a few friends came over and we served the remaining food and opened the gifts we never got to open. Everyone still speaks of that special day. And the good times they all had. To this very day, friends, co-workers and neighbors talk about how close my family and I are. My parents and siblings and Dwight and I are almost inseparable, we have always been and we do plan to remain that way.

The next few weeks we spent getting used to the idea of being married, and I used to say my new name over and over again. I used to write it over and over again also, Mrs. Dwight Alexander. People who had heard that we were married all asked to see my rings, and I would gladly accommodate them, proudly displaying my hand and watching their eyes as my diamonds sparkled for them. While decorating for Christmas last year, my neighbor came over as I was putting garland on my porch and she said "Phyllis, I can't get over your rings, they are beautiful." With my chest poked out, I accepted the compliment graciously. You would think my diamonds were as big as Elizabeth Taylor's, but they are to me because they were given to me out of extraordinary love, during a time when I needed that kind of love, to want to survive. Dwight, helped me to want to fight, so that we could spend our lives together, here and in eternity. As I often look back on all that I have been through, my family was great, but I could not have made it without Dwight, to be there for me and knowing he still wanted to marry me, just as I was. It really made me fight that much more, because I no longer had to go home to a empty house. That song by Luther Vandross really sums this up, the song says "A house is not a home, when you have no one to share it with, no one to hold you tight, and no one you can kiss good night." If GOD had not sent Dwight into my life when he did, my nights would have been unbearable, no one should ever have to go through such a dreaded disease like cancer, alone. Those nights when I was racked with pain ripping through my body, when even the pain medication wasn't working, when I was screaming out for the Lord, begging him to please stop the pain, so that I could get some sleep, if only I could sleep. Dwight was there holding me in his arms, crying along with me, trying to console me. Wishing he could take some of my pain, so I wouldn't have to suffer so. This is what I mean by having someone special there.

Now that the wedding was all over, it was time to get back to the remainder of my treatment. It was now time to start my radiation treatment. So on June 13th, 1994, 1 went in for my first treatment, I was to receive this for seven weeks, going every day, Monday through Friday. My hair had started coming in very good, since the end of chemo. The day I stood before the minister, Reverend Hurst, who also made it a regular visit to come and pray with me, I had a small afro. He and his wife are so special to me. While my hair was in that short afro, I remember being so very proud that I had hair on my head again.

The radiation treatment, Dr. Nichini informed me, you lay on a table with a large machine that looks much like a x-ray machine over you and rays are directed to your breast area. You have to remain very, very still, which is the most uncomfortable part of the whole procedure. You lay like that for about forty-five minutes. After several treatments, I noticed my hair was coming out again, and I mentioned it to both my doctors, and they both replied, it does happen sometime. I said to myself, "Oh, Phyllis it's happening again:In all my literature and in speaking to other patients, I had never heard of anyone's hair coming out from radiation treatment. But mine did, it was just my luck. This time I wasn't as upset as I was when it happened the first time. For the remainder of my treatment, I used to sit and just watch the other patients waiting to be called. And realized that one thing for sure, the BIG C did not discriminate, for there we sat next to each other, black and white and we were all fighting for our lives. There in that radiation suite, we were all brothers and sisters. If we weren't outside of there, we were inside of "that" suite. The technicians there were very nice also, they constantly reminded me to keep very still. My left am was lifted up over my head, so that the rays could penetrate to my underarm, where the lymph nodes were removed. The rest of your body is covered with a lead sheet to protect the areas not being treated. But I believe it did penetrate, besides my hair going completely bald again, that treatment wasn't bad at all.

It was time to go on our honeymoon now, everything was completed finally, all my treatments were done. It was time to take a rest, so I called and made reservations to go to the Poconos Mountain. We rented a white small car, because we had a station wagon and I was not about to travel in that. Remember, I was celebrating my life. We had a cabin, because it was more secluded and I didn't want to stay in the hotel, we had always stayed in hotels. I wanted to try new and different things now.

The cabin was off in the woods because we wanted to be alone and Dwight said that I would get much needed rest in the cabin. I was so excited about being there, that I didn't get much rest, I was alive. At night while he slept, I would caress his face and say "you, my dear husband, needed this trip as much as I did, he could now sleep without hearing me moan in pain. And I said to the Lord, "Thank you Dear Lord, for sending my prince. I was surprised at the size of the cabin, it reminded me of a ranch style house, with everything on one floor. When you entered there was a sunk-in living room, with a beautiful fireplace, but not as pretty as the one we had home. It was a full living room, with color TV and beautiful furniture, then you stepped up into a large bedroom with two double beds, which we only used one, it was our honeymoon, and besides, we had never slept apart before, except when I was in the hospital. There was also a refrigerator, and we were delighted because we had brought a bottle of champagne with us. Next to the bedroom was a jacuzzi whirlpool. I couldn't wait to get into that, and just lay back and unwind, we had fun in there.

Last but not least, this is what really made me get the cabin there was a swimming pool right inside our cabin, a heated pool. The pool lead out to a terrace, I could not get over the fact, that we had a pool, which was built down in the ground, and encased with glass sliding doors, simply magnificent. I took plenty of pictures and my co-workers still couldn't believe it. I was very self conscious at the time, about putting a bathing suit on. So this was perfect, no one would see me but my husband, and boy did we have fun in that pool, I felt so at ease, with just us two sharing the pool, so I wouldn't have to think that everyone was looking at me. We went out for all three meals, but other than that we didn't have to leave our room. We stayed for a weekend, and near the end of our trip, we found out that room service was delivered to the cabins. As I look back on it, I realized we had such a fantastic experience, and the memories will last us a lifetime.

A couple of weeks later still reeling from our trip to the mountains we made plans to go to Baltimore to a crab feast, we were enjoying life, and whatever trip came along you can bet Phyllis and Dwight Alexander were there. This was also a weekend trip and I often look at the pictures, of the two of us waiting for the bus, and taking pictures of each other. My sisters tease us because we were dressed alike in two piece short sets, I thought we looked really cool and I overheard another couple saying that they should have kept the plans they had to dress alike also. Remember the radiation had taken my hair out again, so my head was practically bald, but I didn't care I was having the time of my life, like I just started to live. We had a ball there too, I love to dance, but found that I became tired very easily. But I told Dwight to go on and dance because he enjoyed dancing. Also, but only with my sisters or someone in our party. I was jealous of Dwight, because I didn't want anyone to take him away from me. That was insecurity talking, God had sent him to me and if he didn't leave me when I looked awful, he wasn't about to leave me now.

Before I knew it, it was time for an annual trip to the shore, we went to Wildwood, New Jersey, to walk the board walk and to relax on the beach. We had been going for a few years now, my sisters, their partners, their children, my husband and I and my three year old step-son Yohonnon. This time was special to me, and I think I enjoyed it the most out of all the years we had been going. Four glorious days of fun, rest and relaxation. From our balcony, we can see the ferris wheel, and all the lights from the stores on the boardwalk, that's how close we are. At night it is especially beautiful. Usually we have about three rooms right next to each other, but lately we have about six, which is almost the entire top level or top balcony, life was great. And I wanted to get back on track. I wanted to get back to as normal as possible, but I knew my life would never be the same.

The holidays were fast approaching, and I was elated to be spending them with my family. Thanksgiving was spent traditionally at my parents house and I had plenty to be thankful for. The next day Dwight and I had everyone come to our house, I served turkey but we cooked fried chicken, ham, chitterlings and all the trimmings. Dwight also made his special sweet potato pies, mom loves them. We now have our own tradition, that day after Thanksgiving.

This Christmas Eve, was also spent in Church with my mother and sisters but something went through me in church that night and before I knew it, as father was saying mass, I actually felt the Holy Spirit fill my body. And I turned to my mother, she was crying also, she had felt it. The joy, peace and abundance of love, the experience truly overwhelmed me. As I continued to sob, she reached over and hugged me, her embrace, and that of the Holy Spirit, emanated to my very soul.

It was the week between Christmas and New Years, and my family were preparing to attend my cousin Henry's wedding. He is the son of my Aunt Reedie, who prayed with me on the day of the diagnosis. She would call me often as I went through my treatments. He was to be married on New Year's Eve, at the same community center I was married at, when he called me to tell me he was getting married, I suggested the center, because as he was reminded, it accommodated our large family. So my aunt called me for the information and the arrangements were made. I often told Henry I would believe it when I saw it with my own two eyes. But I didn't because a few days before the wedding, I started to come down with what I thought was the flu. I thought that my resistance was very low, because of the stress and strain, that I had encountered. As I lay on my couch, nodding from the over the counter medication I was taking, my chest started to hurt very badly and when I reached up to touch it, the left side, I screamed out for Dwight, who was also nodding in his chair. I screamed out, Dwight, please come feel this. When he reached down to feel it his eyes began to open wide, and when he could speak he said, "do you want to go the emergency room?" I said no, but I realized later that was a serious mistake. I knew I should have went, but I was just so very tired of being picked and probed on. I told Dwight that I would call the doctor the first thing in the morning. When I called the office in the morning the doctor told me to come in right away. I did, and as I was waiting to a called, my chest area was getting tighter and tighter. As the nurse walked past me I told her of my unbearable pain she told me to come with her, and I was lead to an examining room. She took my temperature, when she took my blood pressure it was very high. The temperature is what really made her call for the doctor. It was actually 104 degrees, and I was going to faint any minute. The doctor came and checked me over and when he felt my chest area along with the high fever, he turned to the nurse and said "I want her admitted right away." I told the nurse that I would have to leave word for my husband, and she immediately took me to the nurse's station and there I was given a phone to use. My parents were called, because I could not think of where my husband was working that day. My poor mother was so upset, she told me later that after the call, she turned to my father and said, "how much more can she take?" and my father answered, "she is very strong, she will get through this like all the other trials, with our prayers."

My family are very religious people, my dad and uncles and aunts all went to Catholic school. St. Peter Claver, is the school we heard about so much growing up. We often heard about my father and my uncle Bobby, being alter boys, and them learning Latin, which they said was very hard, and I agree. After my mom married dad, she loved the Catholic Religion so much, that she took lessons and became a better and more religious person than all of us put together.

They admitted me again to the same hospital, that I had the mastectomy done, and what memories it brought back to me as I was taken to my room. After all my lab work was done, the doctor and his residents came to my room and informed me of the results. In laymen terms, so that you can understand what the doctor told me, because of all the medical jargon that they speak, that's why as you may have noticed, I wrote this book in very simple words, so that everyone reading it will know exactly what they are reading. I was told that my body had rejected the expander, implanted in my chest to stretch the skin, so that it could accommodate the permanent implant. There was a serious infection going through my body, and that was the cause of the high fever and the hardening of the skin on my chest. Before he could speak again I said take it out, the doctor said that's exactly what we are going to do. He said, "it does happen sometimes." I also was told that I would have to be on around the 'clock antibiotics, they had already started to give them to me through my I.V., I wanted to know how long I would have to be in the hospital this time, and was told probably three days or so, but they would know for sure after surgery. After the doctors left, I said to myself, DEAR LORD, I guess these are some more of my trials and tribulations, and I know you haven't brought me this far to leave me now. As I waited to be taken down, and waited for my husband to come, I remember thinking, why didn't I just have the mastectomy done, and after I healed, just go with the prosthesis, which I now have and it is very comfortable, and looks so natural.

My mother and husband arrived to kiss me, and to say that I would be fine, but I already knew that. I said to them as I was being wheeled out of the room, here I go again, and that the two of them were always there with me. Dwight told me later that my sisters had

69

just missed me when they arrived, we were always there for each other, because that's the way we were raised, and the love we have for each other. By now when I got to the operating room, I knew what to do, I was an old pro at it, The next thing I remember, was the nurse calling out to me, to wake up and all had went well. I was very cold and very shaky just like the former surgery. Did they take it out was the next question I asked, "Yes" she answered. I dozed off again, and when I came to, I wanted to see my family, and the nurse answered, soon. When I returned to my room, the only person I remember seeing was my husband, but I was very groggy and went off to sleep. The following day, I was awaken by the nurse on the morning shift, and she needed to get my vital signs, and when she took my temperature, I asked her if it went down, she said, a little, but you still have the infection in you. The doctors came around later that morning and told me everything had went as planned, and that I would continue on the antibiotics for at least another three or four days. He informed me that it was very serious, and that I did right coming as soon as I did. He said that I really should have come in the emergency room that night, like my husband had suggested. I remained in that hospital for five days. The next couple of days, I was in unbearable pain, as I was trying to reach for the cord to call the nurse for more medication for the pain into the room came my cousin, DEE DEE, as we call her she is from California, and she came in from LA to attend her brother's wedding. With her was my aunt Reedie, I cried when I saw them. I just broke down and cried, I hurt so bad, they both reached down and hugged me, saying you will be alright, the worse is over now.

It was New year's eve when I woke the following morning. I became very sad when I realized it was my cousin's wedding day and I wouldn't be able to attend. I knew he understood that my health was more important. But never the less, I wanted to be there. He was one of the few cousins that called to see how I felt, he called me very often to offer support, when I was ill. My cousin Gator, as we call him, also called to lend support, we went to grade school together and also remained close through the years. Later that day, my husband came and spent the day with me, and he asked what we were going to watch on TV that night, And I said to him "Aren't you going to the wedding?" and he answered "No, I'm staying with you and keep you company.""It's New Year's Eve and I thought we could spend the evening together, before they throw me out." I asked him why wasn't he going to my cousin's wedding and he said I can't go and enjoy myself with you here in pain. I told him to please go and represent the Alexanders and have a good time, for he desperately needed some fun. He stayed with me until a little after visiting hours, because he reminded the nurse of the holiday, and he needed more time with his wife. A couple of hours later, I called the nurse for sleeping pills, I was so sad and lonely, I missed my husband so much. I just wanted to sleep so I wouldn't have to think about everyone at the wedding, having fun, and couples hugging when the New Year came in. The phone ringing woke me up, first I was surprised that the operator let the call come through, but I believe she had a big heart, and really understood what it must be like to be in the hospital on a night like this. It was Dwight, my husband calling to say Happy New Year, and to tell me that he loved me and missed me. Tears were falling all over my gown and I was trying to control them, so I wouldn't make him upset. But to no avail, because I could hear his voice breaking up. I asked where was he and he answered, "I'm at home, I couldn't go without you." Then we both broke up, sobbing like babies, he is my baby. After we calmed down, he said, get some sleep, I'll see you tomorrow, good night. As I was reaching for some tissues, the phone rang again, this time it was my family, calling to wish me Happy New Year. It was my sisters, my mother, my aunts, cousins and even the groom, he said how much he missed me and that everyone asked about me. I felt so good after that.

The Lord knew that I needed to her their voices, and the rest of the night I slept like a baby.

Early that next morning about four, a.m. I was awakened by a lab technician who had to draw more blood, I said to him "I don't know where you are going to get it from." And by now, the port in my chest was removed, and since being admitted to the hospital, I had been stuck numerous times and each time it was harder to find a good vein. I told him he could try, and he did, but no blood, another try, no blood, the third time I said, "that's enough." He called another technician that he said could get some blood from anyone, she was supposed to be very good, She came and told me she would use a very small needle. But she couldn't get anything either. That's it I told them both. "We have to get some blood," there were orders written by your doctor. I told him I didn't care who wrote what, no one was going to touch me. Usually, I am very pleasant, but I had been through enough, most of the nurses told me and my husband how cooperative I was. I was a good patient who could not take anymore. They called the doctor, and in the mean time, I started to get hysterical, I cried out, "enough, I had enough." Right then an older nurse came into the room and said "leave her alone, she can't take anymore." She came over to my bed and sat on the edge and hugged me very tightly. And crying into her ear I said, call my husband I want him to come take me out of this place. The nurse still hugging and caressing me said, "you don't want to call and upset him this time of the night." And I knew I couldn't leave, I was just so overwhelmed at that time. She was a Caucasian woman, hugging this African American woman, who just needed to be held and told at that particular minute that everything was going to be alright. My tears soaked her uniform as I held on to her, not wanting to let go until my husband came. After that the resident came in and informed me that if they couldn't get blood from my arm they would have to get it up in my neck area. I said no way, so they just documented it on my chart that they didn't draw blood. The next day after I had calmed down and my husband was there, the doctor came and read what happened and suggested that they try again, which they did and drew blood and all was well. As I look back on that night, I still remember that nurse's gentle touch, and soothing voice speaking to me, and I believe she was sent by GOD as my guardian angel. I know my guardian angel is always with me, because sometimes I can feel her presence. And I know that nurse was truly an angel of God, for she was right there when I needed her the most, and only GOD knows when is the best time for each of us.

The day finally came, when I would be going home, if my temperature stayed down, and all my lab work continued to look as good as it did, the doctor informed me, that he saw no reason why I could not go home the following day. I was elated after he left my room I got up from bed and walked up and down the hall. I wanted to be strong so that the doctor wouldn't have any reason to keep me. When I could, I called to let Dwight know that I was going home the next day. I also called my parents to let them know.

The next day I called Dwight to let him know that he should stay by the phone, but he said I'll do better than that I will be up there as soon as possible. When he says you can go, we will be out of there together. Sure enough he was there before I knew it, with my dear mom, right along side of him. The doctors entered shortly after and said they would remove the bandages. It was a female resident, who came over and began to unwrap the bandages, and as she did I was turning away, because I didn't want to look at my bare chest. My mother stayed in the corner of the room, but Dwight could see the expression on my face and he knew I didn't want to look. So he came over and leaned down, and took my hand and said, I will look at it first, but I had mixed emotions about my husband seeing the ugly scar, and the empty space that remained. Dwight spoke up and said, hey doc, you guys do a real good job, they all nodded and agreed that the surgery had turned out pretty well. A new bandage was applied, and I was given instructions how to care for the wound and when I should go for follow-up. And I was also told, that if my temperature went back up again to return immediately to the emergency room. That would have meant that I still had some infection somewhere. That's why it is so important to get mammograms, and to do those self examinations, because if the lump is found early enough you may only have to get a lumpectomy. That is also why you should get a baseline mammogram done at forty, which I didn't because I thought forty-five or even fifty was early enough. But that's not true, it is a debate going on about when a woman should get her first one done, I still believe if there was more awareness at that time, I would have had it done at forty and maybe I would still have my breast. This book is to enlighten women to the fact that we need to do everything we can, to help ourselves to be aware of our bodies, until there is a cure found.

It is a brand new year now, 1995, and I felt like a brand new woman. The remaining follow-up visits with my doctors, I informed them all, that I was ready to return to work. After getting a clean bill of health from them all, I returned to work in March of 1995. I was out of work for about fourteen months and couldn't wait to get back. You see, I have been working since I was fourteen years of age. My mom took me to center city, where you received your working papers. I felt so grown up. We come from a family of working people, my father worked two jobs, and my mother did day work, to keep all my sisters and brother in catholic school. So all of my siblings started work early, it is instilled in us to work. I really did enjoy my work, as pediatric medical records clerk, I liked talking to the children when they were afraid of all the shots. And I would decorate for them for all the holidays, but Christmas was special, I would really do it up then. So that is why I was anxious to return. My birthday is March 28 and I went back to work March 30, to a surprise welcome back and birthday celebration combined. The doctor and my co-workers had went out of their way to give me a beautiful party. I have plenty of pictures to always look back on. As I walked into the room where it was given, they all shouted surprise, and I was so overwhelmed, that I broke down. I was so happy to see them all for I knew that I had looked death in the face. And there was a strong possibility that I may have never seen them again. I was overjoyed. Before the diagnosis, it was very hard for me to cry, I just didn't cry that easily. But now, I'm very emotional, and find myself crying quite often, even watching a sad movie on TV Dwight often says he noticed it also but didn't want to say anything for fear it too, would upset me. My brother teases me all the time saying, I remember when you were my strongest sister, I said to him "I still am, because you have to be strong, very strong to fight and survive cancer.' So to my dear brother, who I love dearly, I have always been strong but when you come that close to dying, you do become very emotional. The sad things that you hear in this world today, trigger off a rush of emotions, that take me back to the most sad days of my life, which happens to be my bout with Cancer. I'm reminded of the fact that ALMIGHTY GOD has brought me a long way.

Life was great, I was married, finished with all my cancer treatments, back to work, this was all too good to be true. I say this because of all that had happened the last few years, and I didn't want to be too happy. My suspicions were right, because just a few short months later, I received another test of my faith. I was going about my usual routine of house work when I became very light headed and I started to get the chills. It felt like I was getting a fever, so I climbed the stairs, I thought to myself, I'm going to faint, and I was alone. I made it up and just when I got to my bedroom I grabbed the cordless phone and called my mom. When she answered, I said mom, I don't feel right, something's wrong could you come and bring a thermometer because I can't stand up. By now I have the chills and I'm shaking uncontrollable. I was saying in my mind, "come on mom, come on mom". My mother had hung up the phone, but before she did, she said "mommy is coming hang on". I smile when I think about it now, but by the time my mother and I hung up, it seemed she was coming through the door with the extra key. You have to know my mother andhow she feels about her children. She would swim an ocean, or the sea, getting to us. My father was upstairs when my mom called up to him and told him she was going to see about Phyllis, something was wrong with her child. My dad told me later and we laughed, because he was calling down to her to tell her to be careful, and that he would call my house to see if everything was alright. But my mom was already gone, no one but the GOOD LORD could have stopped her. Dad often says, that he can't be around his children, when we are suffering, because he feels so helpless. He can't stand to see us in any kind of pain. He will get you some help but he can't handle it. He will call and get you help but it won't be him, and all of us siblings know and understand. All of my family say that we act and look just alike, friends often tell us that also. My dad makes me laugh and he is my friend as well as my father. Out of all four girls, I'm the one who will cut up with him constantly, we have that kind of relationship. We call each other several times a day. When my mother finally made it to my bedroom she took one look at her child and said "you are very sick baby, and she touched my body while taking my temperature she replied you are burning up with fever. After she removed the thermometer it read 103 degrees. By now my body was shaking so bad, it had the entire bed shaking, and my mother said I have to get you out of here, you are going into convulsions. She had to get me up on the side of the bed to get me dressed, because the house dress I had on and my underwear were soaking wet. When she got me downstairs, she said I had better call 911 because I was trying to think of a family member who wasn't working. But the two of us just couldn't think at the time. After calling for an ambulance, she thought she better call my dad, so he could let my husband know to come to the hospital. He would know to go to the same hospital I had always gone to. And as the LORD would have it, while my mother was checking home to see it everything was alright, my husband beeped in on the other line, checking home to see if everything was alright. He told my mom that he was very close, about five minutes, as he entered the house running, I said to my mother "I'm going out mom, I'm going to faint." But my husband got to me in time and I was put in the front of the car with my brother-in-law Mike. Dwight and mom were with me once again. They rolled me into the emergency room and that's about all I remember, until later when the doctor told me to wake up. As I opened my eyes Dwight was the first one I saw. I asked where was mom and he told me that my brother-in-law took her home, she looked so tired, and I replied, good she is very upset. The doctor told me that I had a severe viral infection and that when they got me to the hospital my temperature had risen to 104 degrees, I needed to be admitted, and that they needed to ask me some more questions. My Dwight had supplied them with most of the information about the breast cancer and the treatments and all my other surgeries. I believed I stayed in that time about four days, I was a little depressed but who wouldn't be after all I had gone though, that showed that I was only human. I was also given heavy antibiotics and once again, I survived another part of my trials and tribulations.

I can't forget to tell you about all of the nurses on Graduate Hospital surgery floor, during those times. They were wonderful and caring people who went beyond their call of duty. One even changed me to a quiet room when I got a noisy roommate. After being discharged, I wrote a letter to the Administration to commend them for the special nurses they had on staff. I know how it feels to not get the thanks we deserve, especially when we go out of our way to do a great job. I'm speaking from experience, because I've been in the medical field for about twenty years, First working in the operating room for fourteen years, then at the medical center for almost six. We only heard about the negative things that were done, never the good, therefore I wanted it to be known that those nurses made a difference in my life. They shall never be forgotten.

The chest pain that I had been experiencing since my treatments for Breast Cancer had started to get worse, now the shortness of breath, was getting me very nervous. I had mentioned it to my Oncologist and she assured me that it had little to do with my treatments. But I insisted that it did not occur until after chemo, radiation and reconstruction with the implant. As I write this book, it is now coming out that women who had implants during Breast Cancer treatments are now complaining of severe side effects. More and more women are having the implants removed because of hardening of the chest. We women, who had this reconstruction done, did it for or as part of our treatments, not for cosmetic purposes. I was trying to make all of my doctors aware that the symptoms that I had been experiencing were real and that they should take a look at the side effects two or three years down the road. I'm going through a reconsideration appeal with Disability, Social Security, because they are trying to say that my new claim has nothing to do with my Breast Cancer. They have to be made aware of the fact that all the hundreds and maybe even thousands of women by the time this book is out, if it does get published, like me who have been saying it all along. The severe symptoms did not happen all the time, so I associated it with my huge weight gain. But to this day the symptoms are worse and even sitting I have them. When I mentioned weight gain to my doctors, they seem to believe that it wasn't all attributed to the medication. I knew it was because before the diagnosis I was no slenderella, but I was an average size for my bone structure. So I went out and bought a Physician's Desk Reference book, which explains the medication that I remain on, side effects are weight gain, and water retention. I know what you are thinking that I should be grateful to be alive. I am, but I started to think the doctor was correct. But no matter what diet I went on, I would only lose a pound or two, I could starve myself, and I still wouldn't lose that weight. In my mind I thought that the weight gain was the cause of the shortness of breathe and the severe chest pain. Some days at work I could hardly walk down the hall, without holding on to the wall. Once a patient even stopped and asked if I needed help. This alarmed me, and my co-workers were now noticing that something was really wrong with me, and suggested that I get a referral to see a cardiologist. Which I did, he suggested a Cardiac Catherization, because it was getting so bad, I couldn't even walk a half a block. I had started to walk a few blocks after work, still thinking it was the weight.

In June, I had the procedure done, the doctor gives you local anesthesia and then a catherater is inserted into your groin area. It travels up into your heart and they can see the picture of it, as it moves about around the heart. I could also watch the screen, it was fascinating. The results were, that there was no blockage, and everything looked fine, Thank God, but it still didn't find the cause for my discomfort. Then one day I ran into my cousin who suffers with Asthma and I told her of the outcome of the heart procedure. She right away said you should go to the doctor and tell them you want to be checked for asthma. I said to her you must be crazy, Asthma at my age, forty five years old? She said just try it. I went to my PCP and asked her to order a Pulmonary test and I told her what my cousin suspected. I had stress test done prior to the heart procedure, and I could not get through it. I shouted out "please get me off, I feel like I'm having a heart attack, The nurse stopped the treadmill. My heart rate had went through the roof. Now as I was blowing into this machine, during the Pulmonary test, again I could hardly get through it. My results from that test was given to my PCP and I made an appointment to see the Asthma/Allergist, Dr. Caleb who had an office down the hall from my office, She verified from the test results that I had asthma. A skin test was ordered which came back that I was allergic to many foods and that my main trigger to induce an allergic reaction, which would bring on an asthma attack was dust, and dust mites. I worked in medical records and dust was everywhere. That's what kept me in so much distress, so the doctor started me on allergy shots. First I was getting them once a week then twice a week and then up to three times a week, it had gotten that bad. The shots were starting to work because I wasn't in as much discomfort as before the shots. Then in October I would come to work early as usual and would be fine, and then after being in the dust for a couple of hours I would start to feel the tightness in the chest, and the shortness of breathe coming on, I started to pant, and I pulled out my inhalers I was given. I was doing my maintenance inhalers but to no avail, I needed the emergency inhaler more and more. It would get so bad I could hardly breathe and I made it to the nurses's station. Once there Nancy or Maryann, whoever was working the station that day, I believe it was Nancy immediately put me on the nebulizer, breathing machine, I would be sent home for a couple of days. One attack was so bad they were about to send me to the nearest hospital because the P.A. could not hear any air moving in my lungs. I would come back to work and the whole process would start over again. On one of my follow up visits to Dr. Caleb she suggested that I purchase a nebulizer for home which I did and this kept me from going to the emergency room all the time. Except for the night my machine just wasn't doing what it normally does. My husband took me to the ER and there I was put on again and then was given some steroids, and a prescription for a steroids pack to take for the next seven days. By now I had purchased a couple of air purifiers for my office and for home, to clean the air in both places. Dr Caleb also ordered blood work done because she believed I also had a condition called Angioedema. This means my body no longer gets rid of inflammation the way it had before. The results came back that I indeed had this condition, and it had plenty to do with the way I had been feeling, and still do, even today. By now it had gotten to the point I couldn't work anymore so Dr. Caleb suggested taking me out of what was triggering these numerous attacks. She decided that I should go on a medical leave of absence for at lease six months. I was constantly in an asthma attack because of the high incidence of dust in my work area. Some co-worker asked my doctor how could I be put out on leave and not her, I told her she should have directed her to me. For I would have asked this person if she also had gone through chemo, radiation to the lung area and also had she gone through breast reconstruction surgery, with an implant put in and then a couple of months later have it taken out because of a severe infection and severe hardening that if left untreated it could have killed her, I don't think so. That's exactly what I meant about true friends and true Christians because true friends would have never thought to ask the doctor such a ridiculous question. Weeks after that I also went through a viral infection. The asthma I have is severe and chronic due to all the trauma to my lung area, she would never want to go through all I've been through and continue to suffer with. I pray that she never has to see just what exactly I'm speaking of. Each time I go through one of these attacks I say to my husband and to myself GOD, don't let me make it through breast cancer treatments and now let me die from a severe asthma attack.

I applied for Social Security Disability benefits in October when I went out on leave, but as my condition continued to deteriorate, my doctor and I agreed I could no longer work, she wrote a letter to SSI and to my manager and to the personnel department to inform them of the situation and that I should apply for total disability for an indefinite period of time. And recently I was sent a letter stating that because the breast cancer was in remission I was no longer considered disabled. But I am in the process of appealing it because when I filed the claim in October, I stated that I now have respiratory problems and beside the fact I sent them a copy of the letter that the doctor who had been treating me wrote them. And if I have to get my lawyer to step in I will, I have been working since I was fourteen years old and I paid into the system that is now trying not to pay me when I need it. Everything triggers my asthma now, if it's too hot, too cold, too windy, certain odors, and my peak flow, which measures your lung capacity, is always in the danger zone. Most days I can't breathe so I stay inside under my air purifiers, which help somewhat.

So GOD and my wonderful husband Dwight inspired me to write this book, because I wanted to make women aware of this dreaded disease and the side effects that may come down the road years later. Women like me aren't getting those mammograms when we should and a lot of us are dying because we just wait too late. I was truly blessed, because the size of the tumor I could have easily been told it had already spread. Praise the Lord!!! It was a miracle that I lost my breast instead of my life. So I want to help get out the word to maybe spare one, just one woman of having to lose a breast, or her life.

In March of 1997, I was enrolled into a HMO program and there I received a new PCP by the name of Dr. Arthur Williams. This is the doctor who discovered

I had a heart problem, during a visit he heard a distinct heart murmur which was never followed up after the technician called my doctors back in 1993 to make them aware of it. Dr. Williams right away ordered an ekg. The ekg indeed showed that I had an irregular heart beat and that I was having pvc. As he returned to the examination room he had a look of great concern on his face, he went on to say that he did not like the look of my results and immediately gave me referrals to have a echocardiogram done at Graduate hospital ASAP. He mentioned to me that he couldn't believe that the other doctors did not follow up on such a condition. I told him I had a doctor that was concerned about the problem and gave me nitroglycerin to put under my tongue when I had an acute attack. This was when I was going through chemotherapy, and he thought it was due to the treatments I was receiving. My appointment for the test was scheduled for the next day because the clerk at the clinic told the tech at the hospital that the doctor was very concered that the patient may have had a heart attack or about to have one in the near future. The doctor also ordered pulmonary function test for my asthma. That evening I had a bad asthma attack and I told my husband it was probably from all the stress of that day, I had to get on my breathing machine a couple of times that evening. But during the early hours of the following morning I was awakened from my sleep with severe shortness of breath and a fullness in my chest that was very scary. I said to my husband, "Dwight, I want to go to the ER this is not my asthma this time, get me out of here." He helped me get dressed and we arrived at the ER in about five minutes. As we arrived my chest was now very tight and I thought about the pain my dad and others often talked about when going through a heart attack. I remembered to get my husband to get all of my medication to take with us. When we arrived they took me right back after my husband told the nurse he thought I was having a heart attack. A female resident came right over to me and started a history and physical. I told the resident that I had just had several tests done the day before, including the echocardiogram she was getting ready to order. As they were hooking me up to an IV, they were also trying to get in touch with my PCP, I was hooked up to all kind of heart monitors and machines. My husband and I remained in the ER from about six in the am until one thirty. The nurse told us that my PCP was on vacation or a conference and that another doctor from that medical group would be in to see me and also to admit me. I told my husband they were going to admit me because I overheard the conversation when the doctor was calling to get in touch with my doctor. Finally the doctor from the medical group arrived and after speaking with the nurse and doctors he came and spoke with us. He said that after speaking with the team of nurses and doctors and checking the test results that I had taken the day before, I was being admitted because they wanted to continue to monitor me and do more test but from what they had, he said that I had an en-larged heart. As they were wheeling me to the cardiac care unit or telemetry I said to my husband, 'I made it through breast cancer and now I'm going to die from a heart attack or stroke. Then I turned to my husband and he said, PHYLLIS, GOD spared you from breast cancer because HE is not ready for you, you still have a job to do and HE is not ready for you and he was right, my mission is not complete, for I have to get the word out about what GOD can do. You just have to have faith and hope. I remained in the hospital for four days this time and on the day of discharge my cardiologist, Dr. Bruce Berger, and my doctor Dr. Sargeant, came in to explain everything that the test showed. Dr. Berger spoke first, he said in detail that my heart was indeed enlarged and that my heart muscle is very, very thick now and my heart has to work much harder to pump blood through my body, that's the reason for the acute angina attack, and the shortness of breath and the heart palpitations. They were really scary. To accommodate all of this, the heart enlarged itself. He went on to say that this is a condition called Hypertrophic Cardiomyopathy. My pcp Dr. Sargent then spoke up to say it can be treated with medication but that I have to be very careful because I have the same disease that the young basketball player that dropped dead on the court had. He wanted me to know this so that I would do exactly as my doctors tell me to do, and he died because he didn't know that he had this condition. So it was very crucial that I came when I did. Had I not gotten the proper treatment I too would have died. My brother-in-law has a similar condition but the doctors say mine is complicated by asthma and the trauma to my lung area from the radiation. I now wear a nitroglycerin patch and am presently taking alot of a medication, not only for this illness but for Asthma, and Tamoxifen, which is a anti-cancer pill which also complicates my heart condition. The side effects of the Tamoxifen are weight gain and water retention which also makes my heart work harder to try and pump the fluid. Until today I still have trouble with shortness of breath when walking sometimes, and even without out exertion, these days I just stay inside and rest. I still believe all of these diagnosis, HEART FAILURE, ASTHMA, ANGIOEDEMA, ALLERGIES, are all side effects from the chemo and radiation. I have a book about breast cancer survivors and most state that they now have side effects. We are glad to be alive but we just want everyone to know that we are not crazy and that doctors, oncologist can at least admit that there is a possibility that indeed these side effects are a major part of chemo treatment just as mouth sores, stomach nausea, that happen during treatment. Not only oncologist should open their minds to possibilities but also the goverment (SSI DISABILITY) because as I mentioned earlier when I first applied in October of 1996, I was told since the cancer is in remission that I was no longer eligible for benefits but it is all connected. I had none of these conditions until after going through the cancer treatments.

To all my sisters and brothers alike we are forever united through this dreadful disease and should do our best to spread the word to get those mammograms and do the self-examinations. I've always enjoyed helping people when I can, my family can attest to that. But I find some people don't always want help so I back off and pray for them but try, try hard. I pray that this is published, so that anyone out there who needs an ear from someone who has been there, or if you want to cry, my number and address is in the back of the book. I wish I had someone at the time of my treatments who had also lost a breast, to talk and cry with. Elaine was the closest person that I know that had cancer but even she couldn't know the trauma of loosing a part of your body. For you see, she did not have breast cancer, and I shall forever love her for being there to help me with the things she could. Loosing a part of yourself that you were born with was the single most devastating thing to happen in my life, even now with all the illnesses that I'm going through, even heart failure, none can compare.

The following was saved for last; the first time that I actually looked down at the empty space where there use to be a breast, for forty-two years, I began to cry, this disease had taken a part of my body. Only another breast cancer patient could know the pain, the hurt, the sadness that I felt. And remember I was a few months away from being a bride with the man GOD had sent in my life. But GOD knew to send him because GOD knew it wouldn't make a difference, here comes the tears again. I use to lay in bed at night and say "OK cancer, you took my breast, (I had reconstruction and that didn't take) but you will NOT take my life." I used to shout it out To myself I thought, I will win, you made me mad now, my temper took over and at that very moment I decided to fight this cancer. You shall leave my body because I won't let you stay in there, I'm strong and I'm not going to let you take me like that.

So please get those mammograms, do those self examinations, get to know your body, every inch of it, check for changes, and ask your doctors when it's best for you to get your baseline mammograms. In my opinion I believe they should change the age to thirty-five. Don't be like me, I kept thinking I had plenty of time, I was only forty-two and I didn't have to worry until age fifty. I kept saying later, and later cost me my breast and almost my life.

Before I end I would like to thank a few more people that I forgot.

To my niece, Nichelle, thanks for coming to the hospital with the kids to sit with me and thanks for the lovely plant. It really meant a lot to me because I wasn't real sure I was going to make it, my heart is in bad shape and being there hooked up to those heart machines and to see me like that took strong people. I Love you.

To my godchild, Neice Thornton, who typed this manuscript when I couldn't finish it, I wasn't feeling well, Thanks and you were always special to me, that daughter I never had, thanks to my big sister for letting me share you.

And again a very special thank you to my parents, William and Mary Jackson and William Jackson Jr. Business Manager for Local 427, Distric Council #33, who continues to tease me and call me plain old and says it's not the condition it's my age. My soul mate Dwight Alexander who never doubted for a minute that I would make it through all of these illnesses. If he did have doubt, he never let me see it. These four people were with me everyday at the hospital with my heart, they didn't just call on the phone they came to be with me. They were Angels sent to be there for me and they didn't just say the words, they showed me. I LOVE YOU ALL.

So as the title says the healings of breast cancer a physical and spiritual healing of my body and of my soul. For I was truly healed spiritually, GOD and me have a great relationship and this is what HE wanted me to do. Now I know my purpose I still wish that I had children but I am so fulfilled when I help others, and it fills the gap.

GOD bless and keep us all, and REMEMBER WE NEED FAITH TO GET US THERE, AND HOPE TO KEEP US THERE!!!!!!!!!!!!!!

If you need to call 267-269-9953

or write to:

Mrs. Phyllis Alexander
1510 So. Garnet St.
Philadelphia, Penna. 19146
email: alexandphyll@aol.com

I'll be there waiting to hear from you, if it's the good LORD's will.

PS. Just before this manuscript was being mailed, I was called from our community paper, The South Philly Review, the man on the other end of the phone said his name was Randy, and that I was chosen along with three other women to tell about our bouts with BREAST CANCER. The article is for BREAST

CANCER awareness month, I told him it was ironic because I had just finished my manuscript for book publication on the disease to make women aware. My article will be in the October 16th, or October 23rd edition, and I told him I wrote a small article on BREAST CANCER awareness for my church, St. Thomas Aquinas, which will be in my church bulletin for Sunday, October 19th.

God Bless!